Pig in a Muddle

A story by Mira Lobe
illustrated by Winfried Opgenoorth

Oxford University Press

Oxford University Press, Walton Street, Oxford OX2 6DP

Oxford London Glasgow
New York Toronto Melbourne Auckland
Kuala Lumpur Singapore Hong Kong Tokyo
Delhi Bombay Calcutta Madras Karachi
Nairobi Dar es Salaam Cape Town

and associated companies in
Beirut Berlin Ibadan Mexico City Nicosia

OXFORD is a trade mark of Oxford University Press

First published in Germany by Verlag Heinrich Ellermann KG, Munich, 1983
Das quiekfidele Borstentier
© Verlag Heinrich Ellerman KG, Munich, 1983
© English version: Oxford University Press 1983
ISBN 0 19 279783 2

Typeset by Oxford Publishing Services, Oxford
Printed in Germany

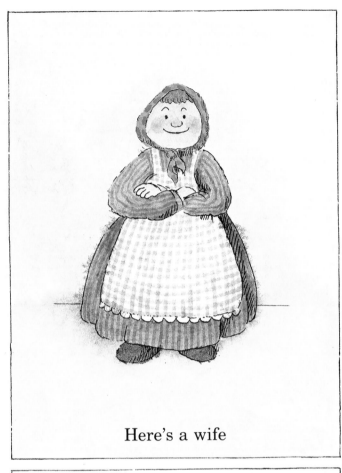

Here's a wife

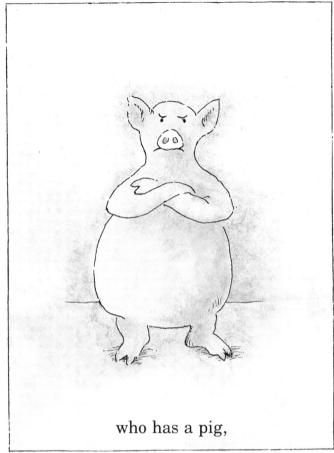

who has a pig,

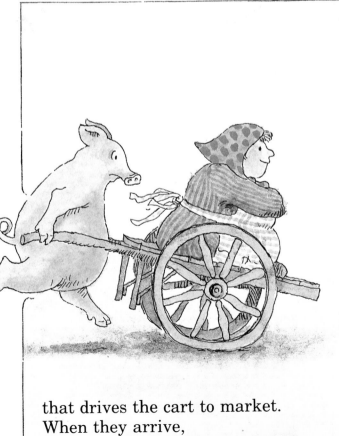

that drives the cart to market.
When they arrive,

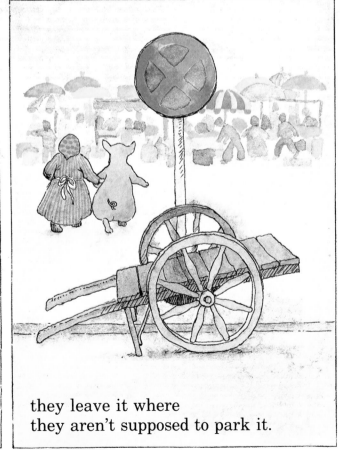

they leave it where
they aren't supposed to park it.

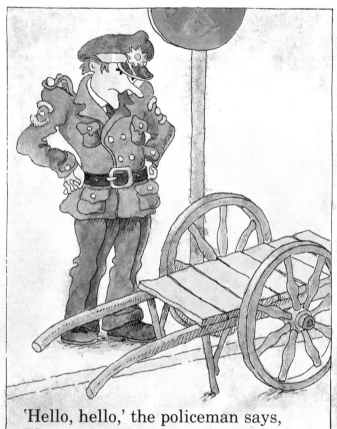

'Hello, hello,' the policeman says,
'You can't leave that thing here.'

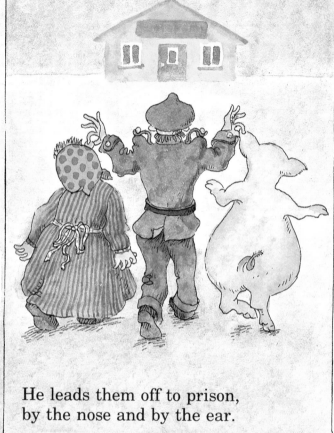

He leads them off to prison,
by the nose and by the ear.

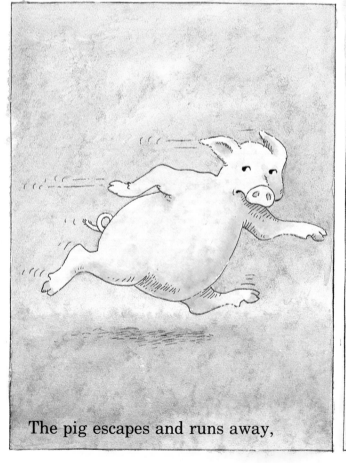

The pig escapes and runs away,

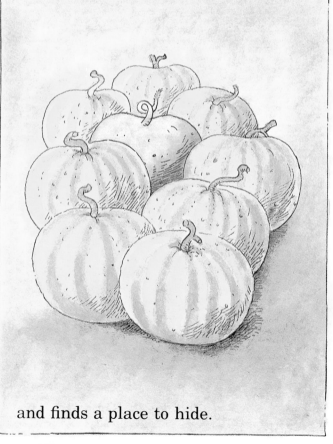

and finds a place to hide.

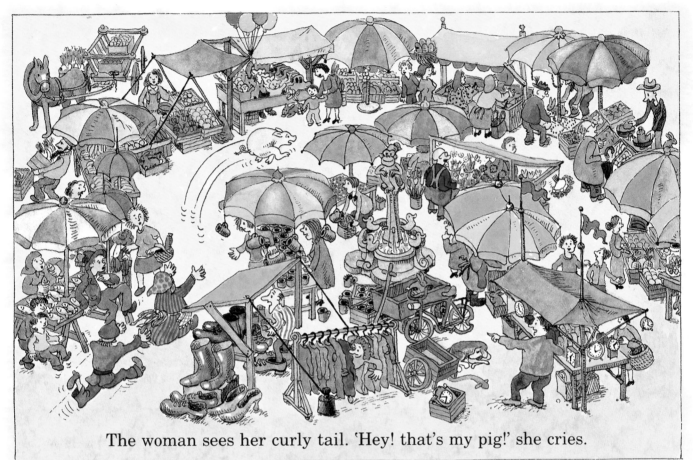

The woman sees her curly tail. 'Hey! that's my pig!' she cries.

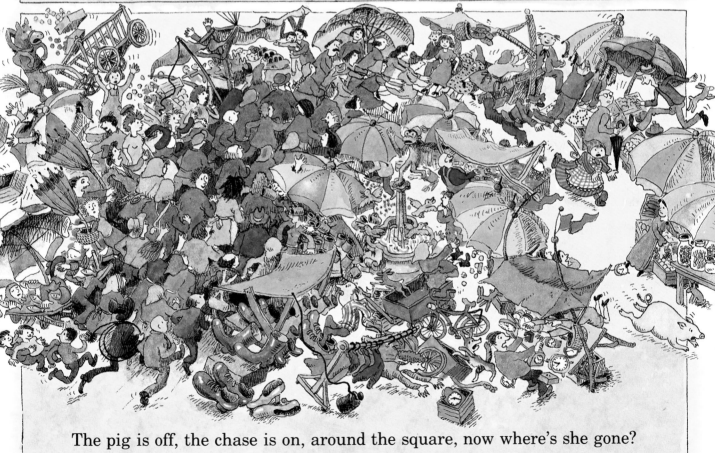

The pig is off, the chase is on, around the square, now where's she gone?

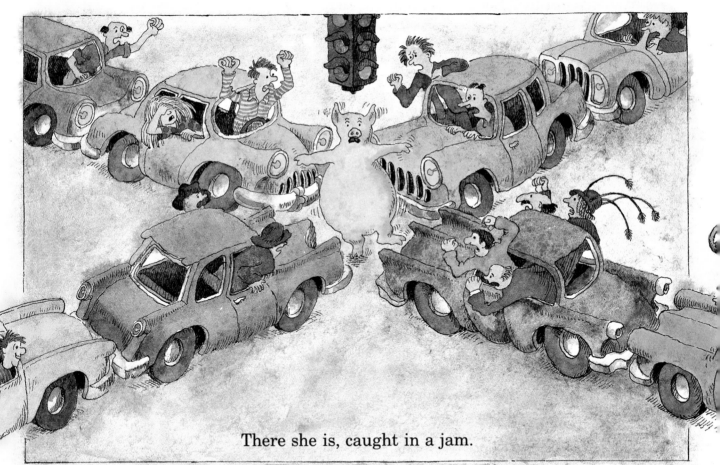

There she is, caught in a jam.

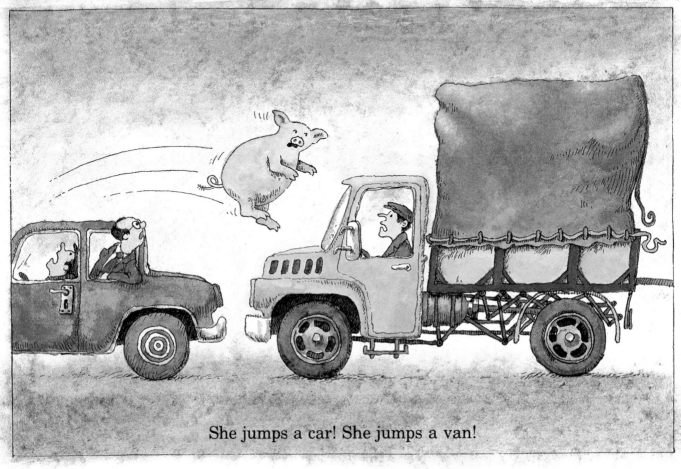

She jumps a car! She jumps a van!

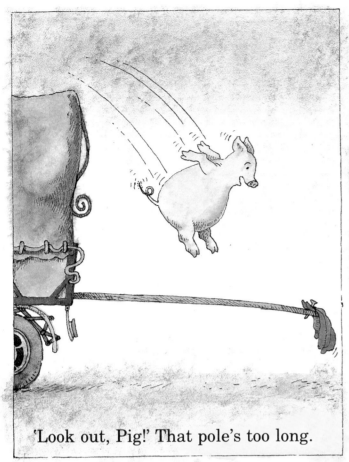

'Look out, Pig!' That pole's too long.

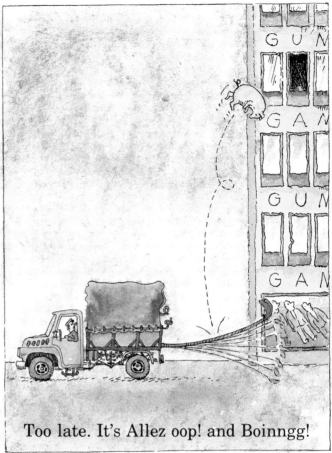

Too late. It's Allez oop! and Boinngg!

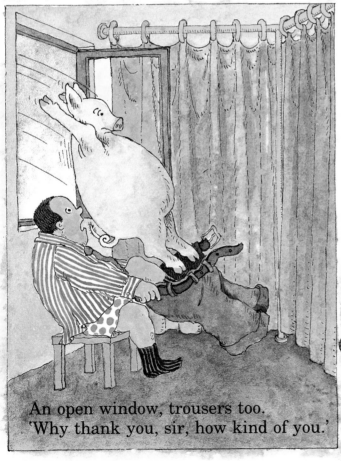

An open window, trousers too.
'Why thank you, sir, how kind of you.'

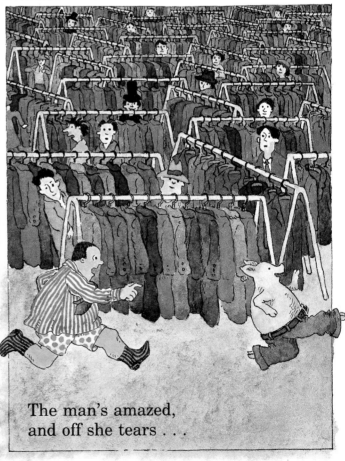

The man's amazed,
and off she tears . . .

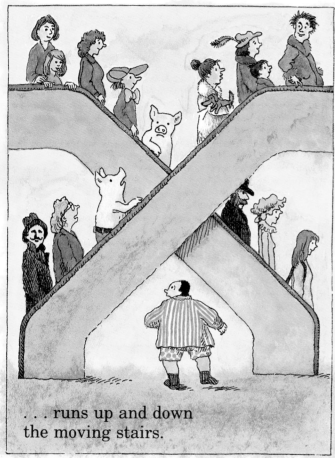

. . . runs up and down
the moving stairs.

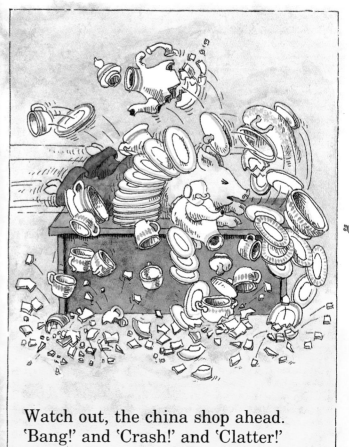

Watch out, the china shop ahead.
'Bang!' and 'Crash!' and 'Clatter!'

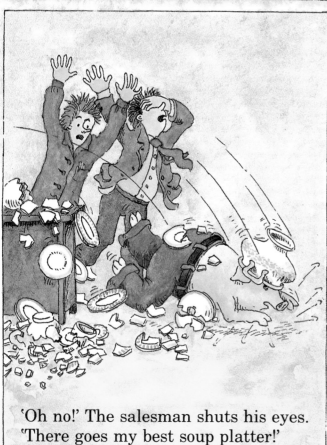

'Oh no!' The salesman shuts his eyes.
'There goes my best soup platter!'

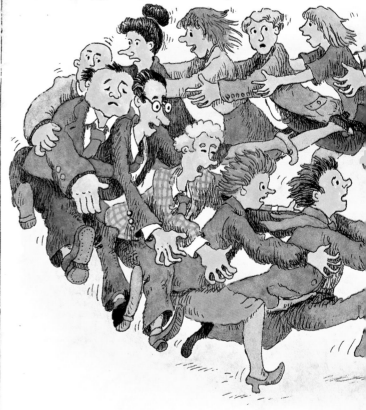

The pig is off, the chase is

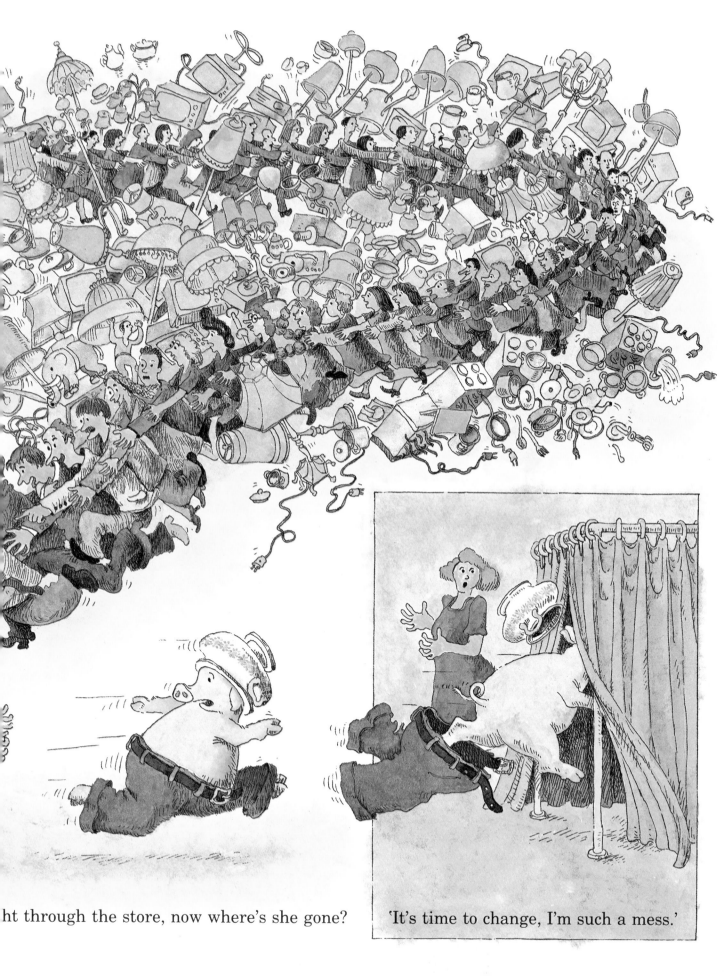

ht through the store, now where's she gone?

'It's time to change, I'm such a mess.'

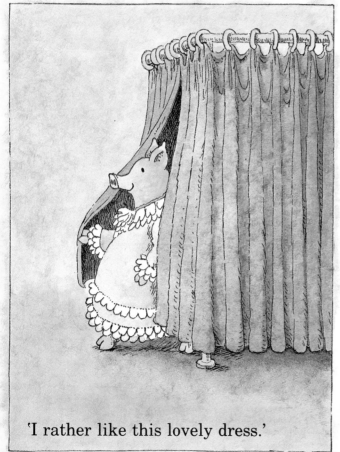

'I rather like this lovely dress.'

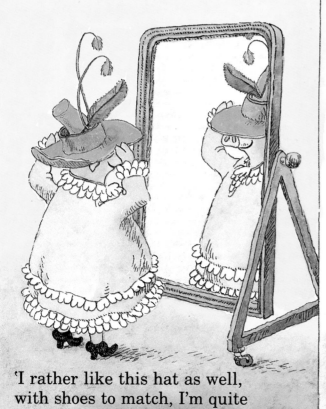

'I rather like this hat as well,
with shoes to match, I'm quite
a belle!'

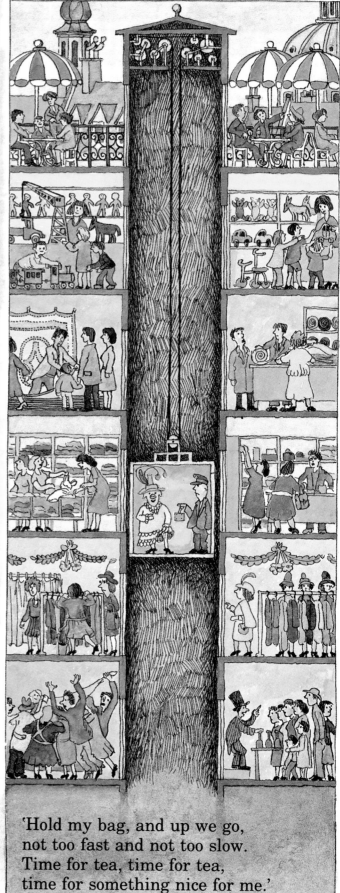

'Hold my bag, and up we go,
not too fast and not too slow.
Time for tea, time for tea,
time for something nice for me.'

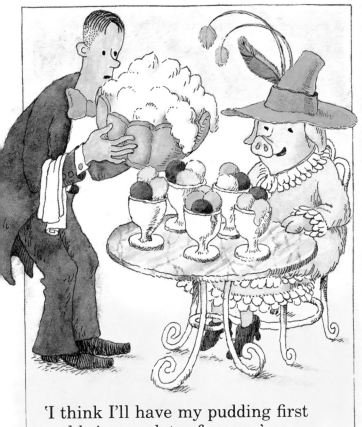

'I think I'll have my pudding first
and bring me lots of cream.'

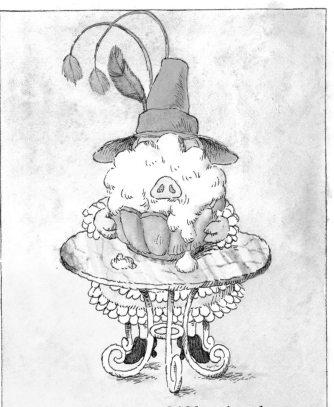

'Slurp' and 'Slop' and 'Glurp' and
'Glop,' a greedy piggy's dream.

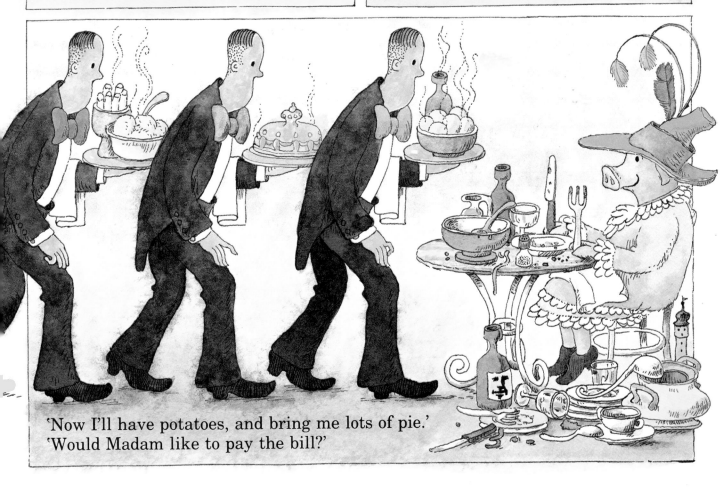

'Now I'll have potatoes, and bring me lots of pie.'
'Would Madam like to pay the bill?'

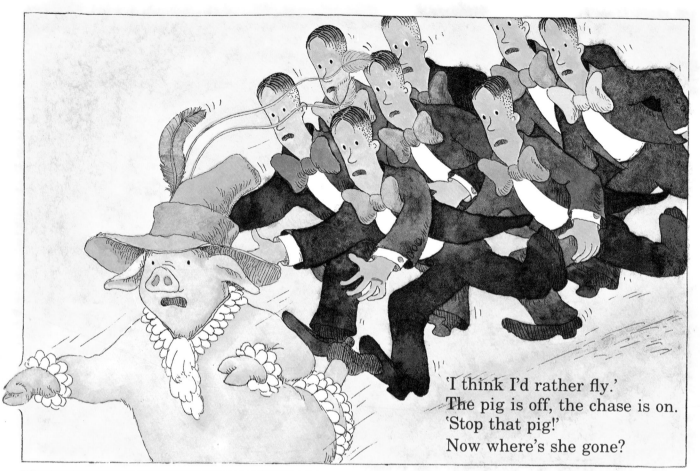

'I think I'd rather fly.'
The pig is off, the chase is on.
'Stop that pig!'
Now where's she gone?

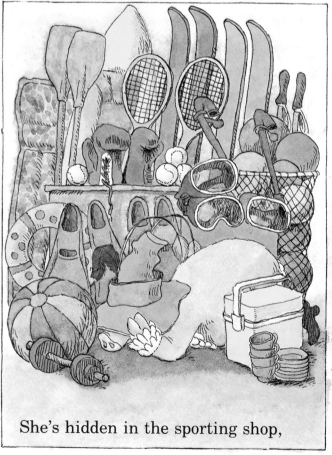

She's hidden in the sporting shop,

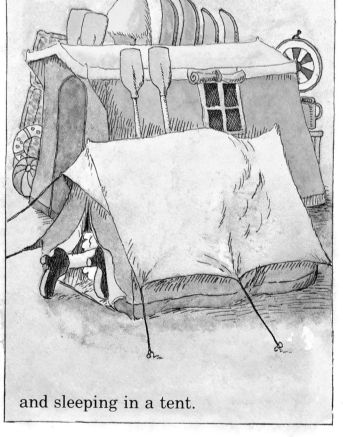

and sleeping in a tent.

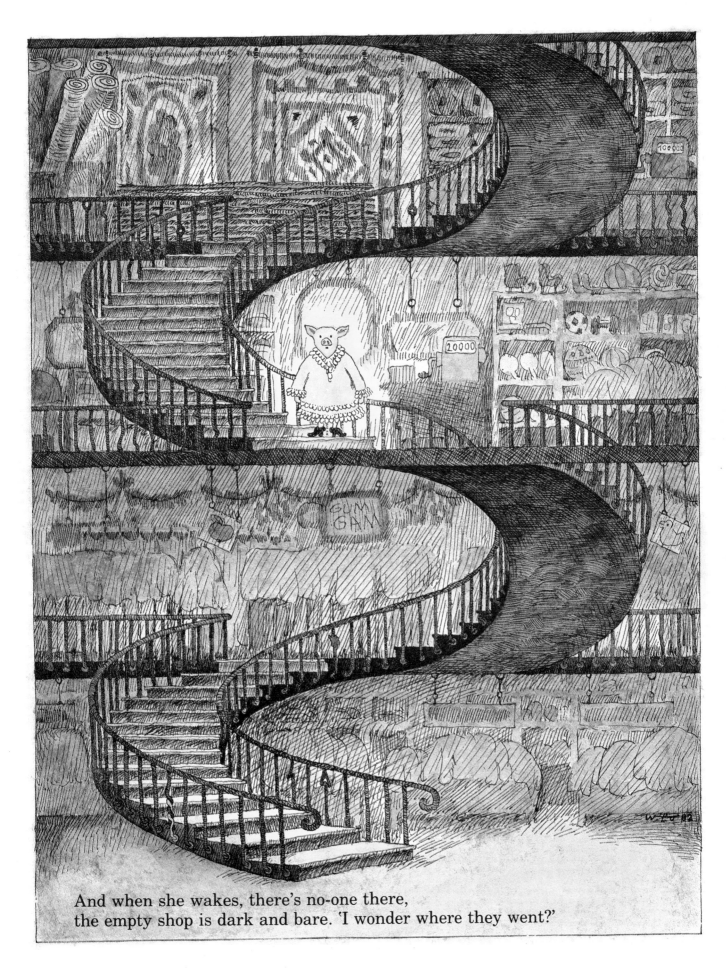

And when she wakes, there's no-one there,
the empty shop is dark and bare. 'I wonder where they went?'

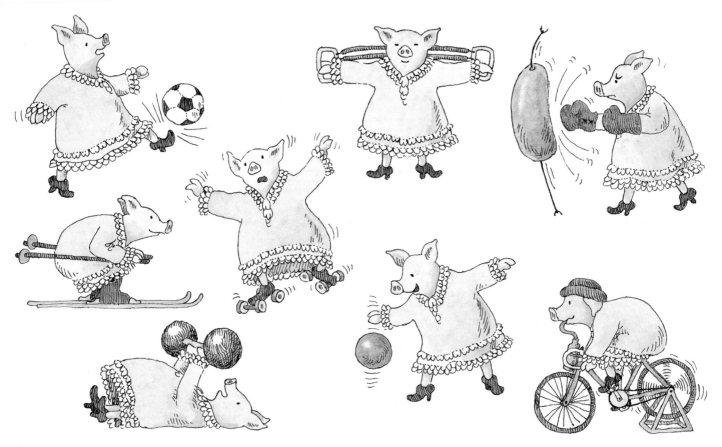

She tries out all the sporting gear . . .

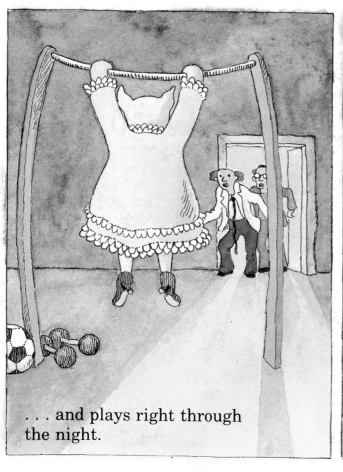

. . . and plays right through the night.

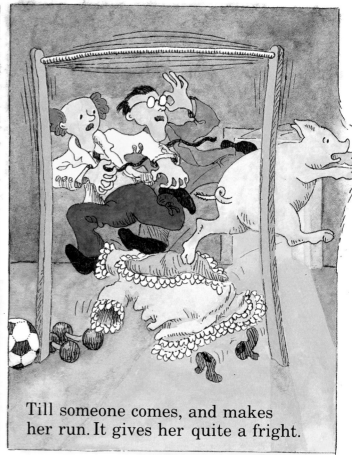

Till someone comes, and makes her run. It gives her quite a fright.

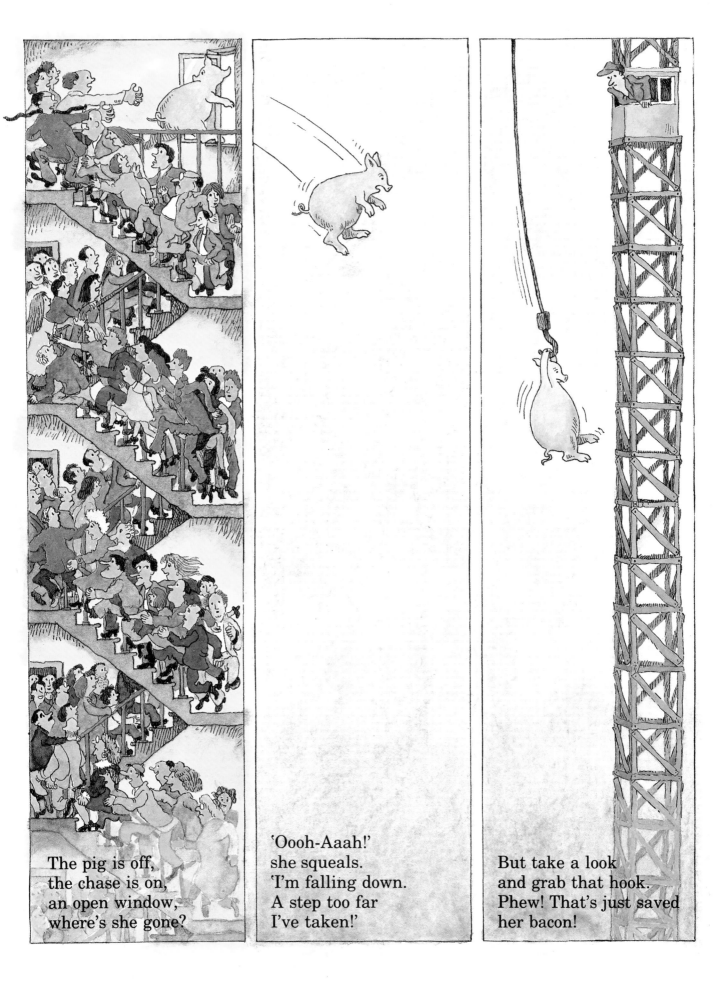

The pig is off,
the chase is on,
an open window,
where's she gone?

'Oooh-Aaah!'
she squeals.
'I'm falling down.
A step too far
I've taken!'

But take a look
and grab that hook.
Phew! That's just saved
her bacon!

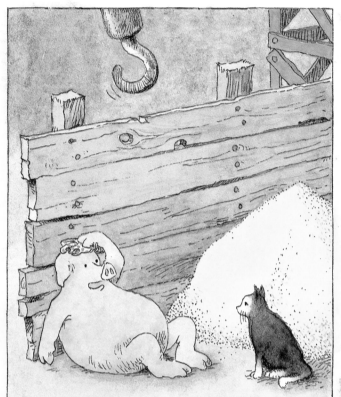

Off the hook, she's fallen flat,
and waiting there she finds a cat.

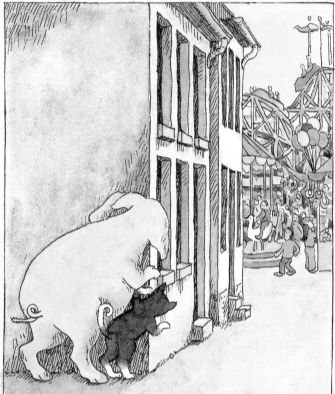

'Don't waste time just lying there!'
'Why don't you take me to the fair?'

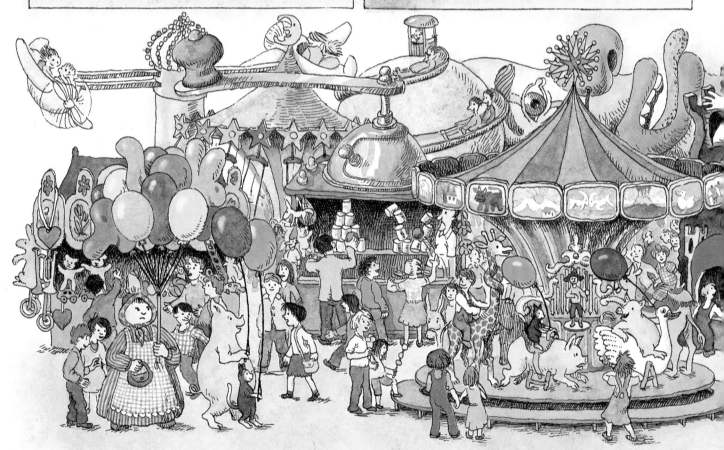

Roll up! Roll up! Let's have a go!

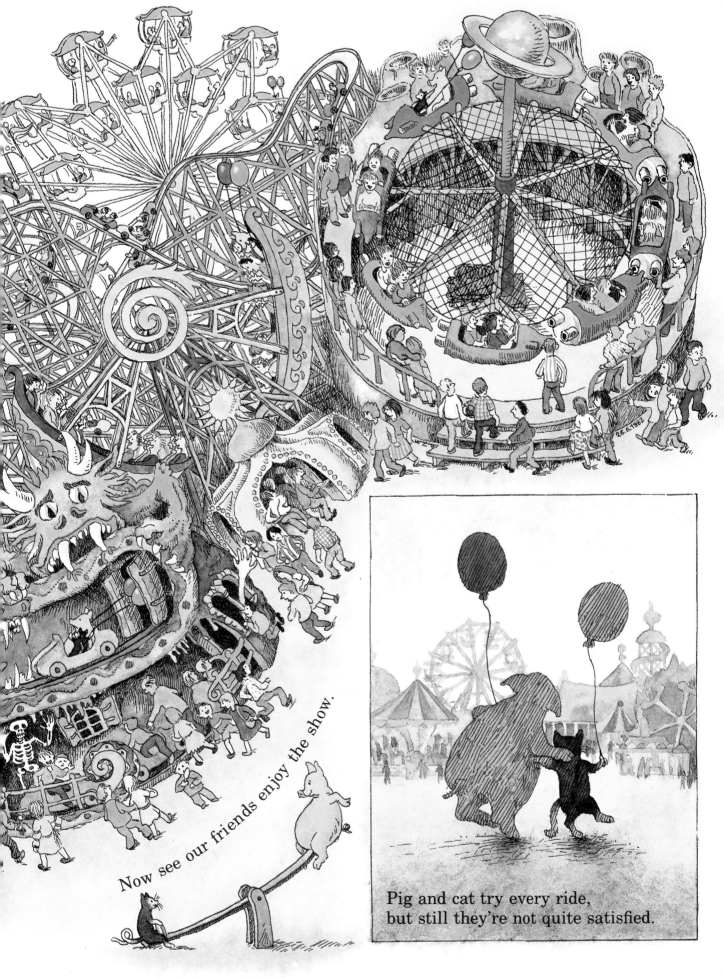

Now see our friends enjoy the show.

Pig and cat try every ride,
but still they're not quite satisfied.

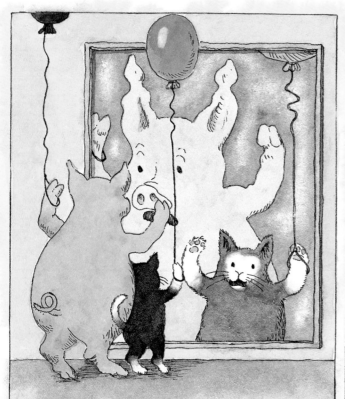

The Hall of Mirrors. What a sight!
'Oh no!' says Pig. 'I'm far too fat.'

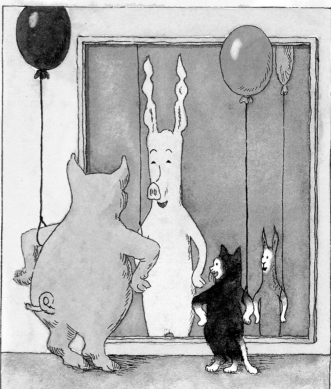

'But over here you look so slight,
and slender, slim and sleek,' says Cat.

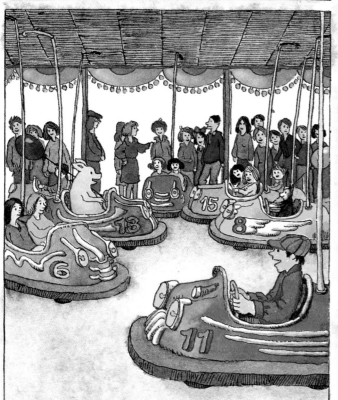

Next they try the Dodgem ride.
Don't go too fast, or you'll collide.

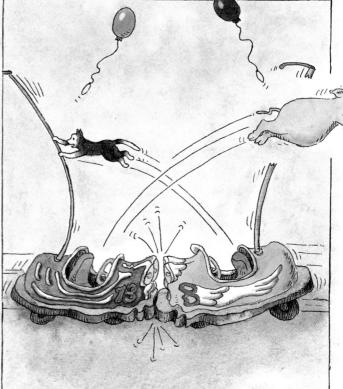

Oh no! They've crashed, the crazy pair.
Just see them flying through the air.

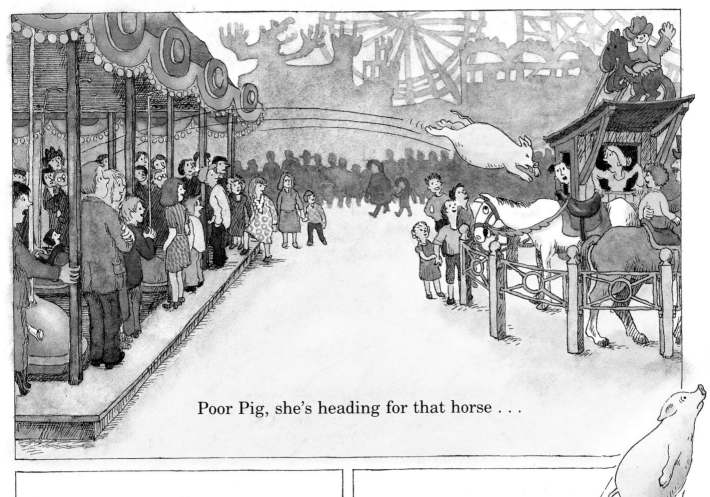

Poor Pig, she's heading for that horse . . .

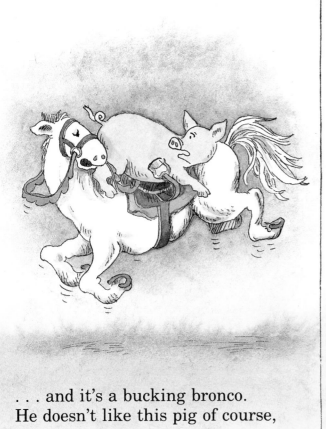

. . . and it's a bucking bronco.
He doesn't like this pig of course,

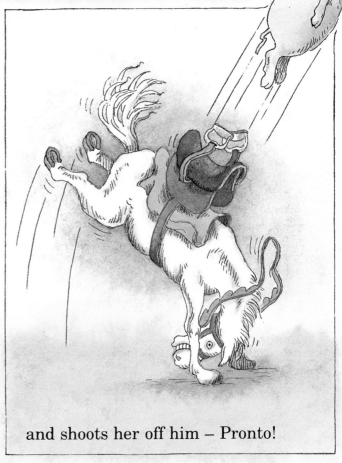

and shoots her off him – Pronto!

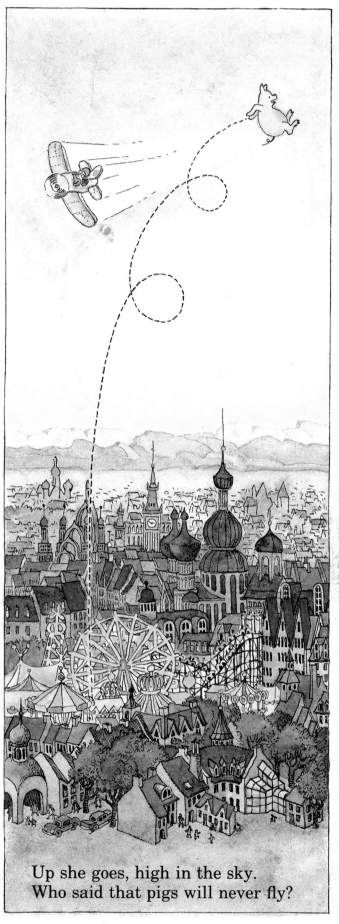

Up she goes, high in the sky.
Who said that pigs will never fly?

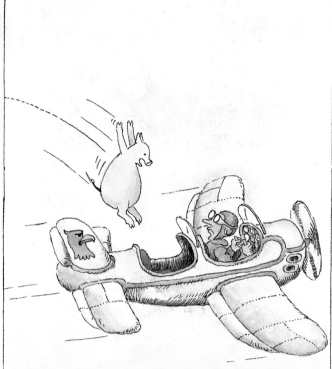

The pilot shouts, she answers him,
'Just passing through?'
'No, dropping in!'

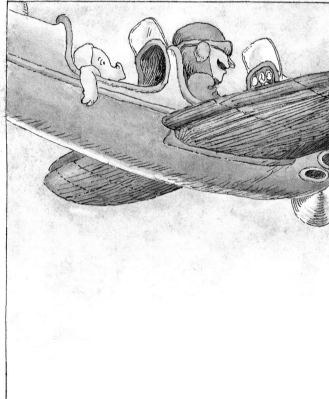

Flying gives our pig the frights,
she hasn't any head for heights.

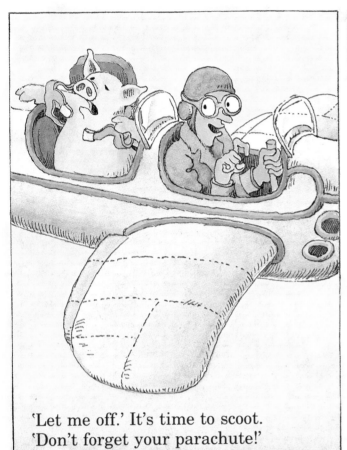

'Let me off.' It's time to scoot.
'Don't forget your parachute!'

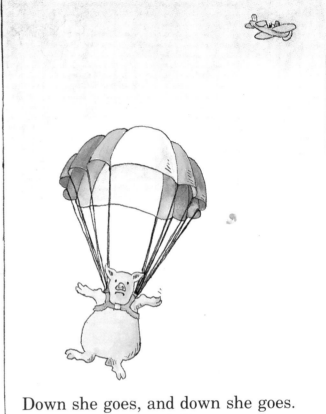

Down she goes, and down she goes.
She floats so gracefully,

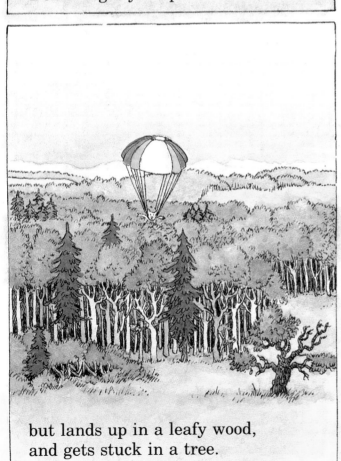

but lands up in a leafy wood,
and gets stuck in a tree.

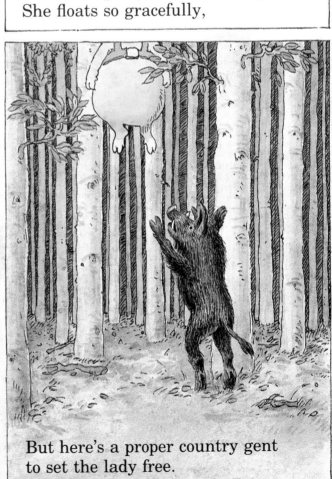

But here's a proper country gent
to set the lady free.

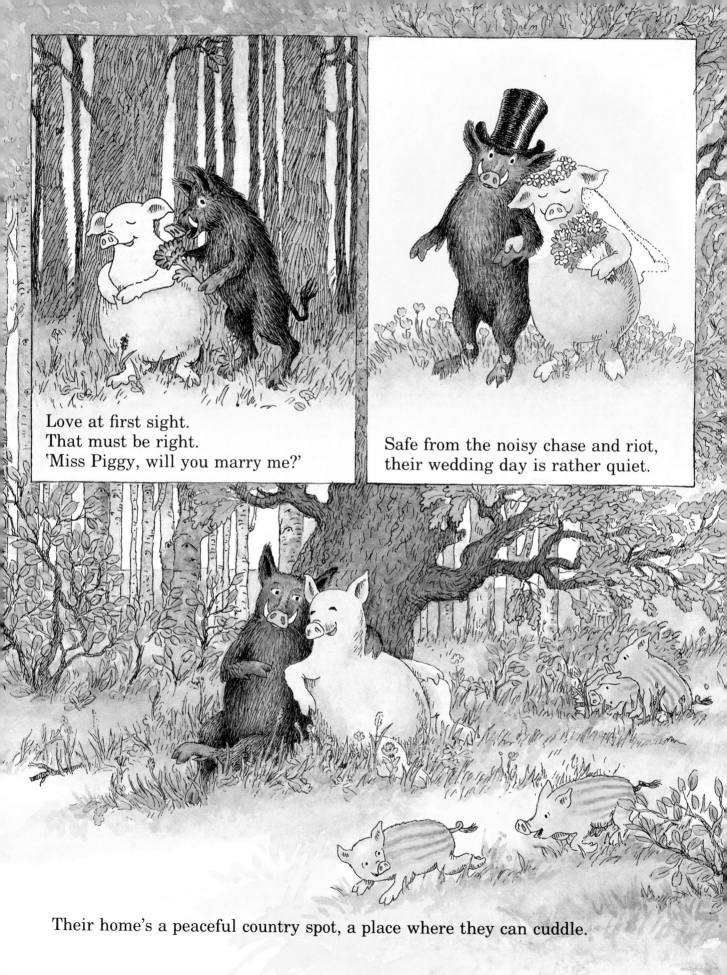

Love at first sight.
That must be right.
'Miss Piggy, will you marry me?'

Safe from the noisy chase and riot,
their wedding day is rather quiet.

Their home's a peaceful country spot, a place where they can cuddle.

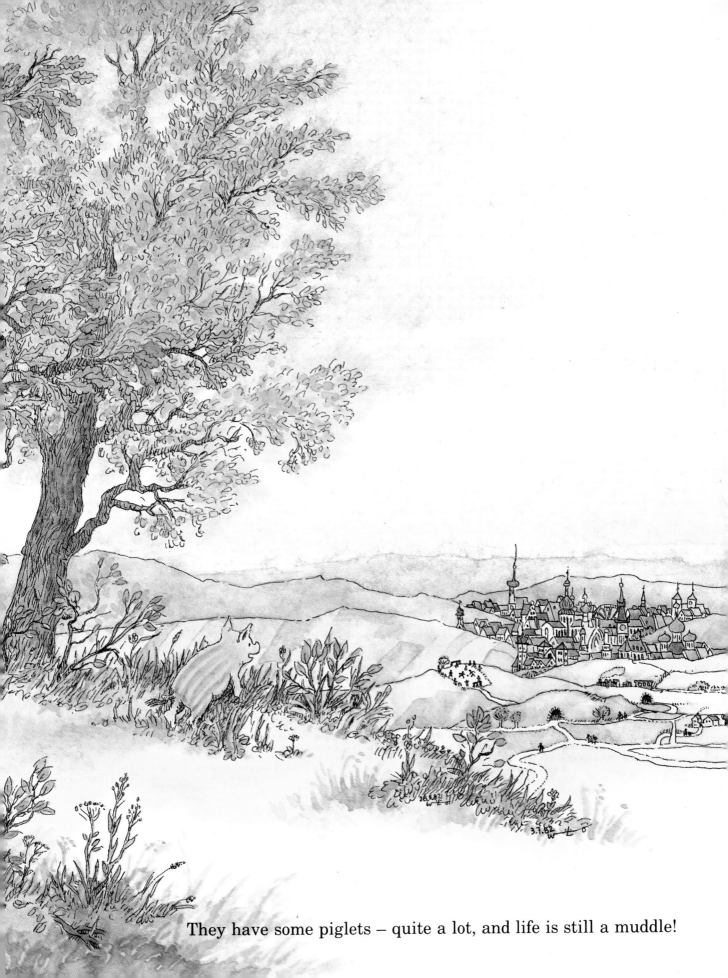

They have some piglets – quite a lot, and life is still a muddle!